THE LITTLE BOOK OF
REIKI

THE LITTLE BOOK OF REIKI

An Hachette UK Company
www.hachette.co.uk

Vie Books, an imprint of Summersdale Publishers
Part of Octopus Publishing Group Limited
Carmelite House
50 Victoria Embankment
LONDON
EC4Y 0DZ
UK

www.summersdale.com

Printed and bound in Poland

ISBN: 978-1-80007-684-6

This FSC® label means
that materials used for
the product have been
responsibly sourced

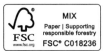

Substantial discounts on bulk quantities of Summersdale books are available to corporations, professional associations and other organizations. For details contact general enquiries: telephone: +44 (0) 1243 771107 or email: enquiries@summersdale.com.

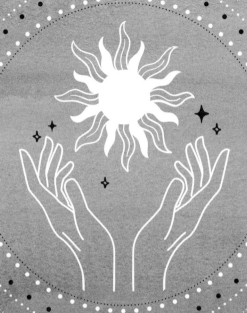

THE LITTLE BOOK OF
REIKI

STEPHANIE DRANE

Disclaimer

Neither the author nor the publisher can be held responsible for any injury, loss or claim arising out of the use, or misuse, of the suggestions made herein. Always consult your doctor before trying any new complementary therapy or if you are worried about any of the side effects.

CONTENTS

INTRODUCTION

Have you ever wondered what Reiki is? You may have heard people talk about its power to change your life for the better, as well as help with physical ailments. But perhaps you've been uncertain how to bring this positive energy into your life.

Well, now is your chance. This book will tell you everything you need to know about Reiki so you can embrace its benefits. You will discover the history of Reiki, learn its principles and understand how they can bring about harmony. As you work through this book, you will learn the hand positions, methods for self-Reiki and suggestions for the many ways you can use Reiki to enhance your life. It will help you access its gentle, reassuring strength whenever you need it.

Once you have made a connection with Reiki it will always be there for you, whether you turn to it daily or once in a while. Use this book as a guiding force for familiarizing yourself with the methods and principles of Reiki and revisit the information whenever you need to. Read on to discover how to create your own unique relationship with this precious gift.

WHAT IS REIKI?

Reiki healing is a beautiful, inclusive complementary therapy that brings balance, peace of mind and well-being to your body, mind and spirit. In this chapter, you will learn how it draws on the universal energy recognized in many religions and spiritual traditions.

A BRIEF HISTORY OF REIKI

Reiki was developed in Japan by a Buddhist monk called Mikao Usui, who was born in 1865. Legend has it that Usui experienced a moment of spiritual enlightenment while meditating alone on a mountain. The story goes that he stubbed his toe on the way home. When he put his hands on his sore toe, the pain vanished and he discovered that he could heal. This was the first of four miracles that he supposedly performed on his way down the mountain.

Although it isn't clear how true this story is and many of the facts are lost to time, we know that Usui was a very spiritual man who taught his healing methods to others, who called it "Usui Do" (the Usui method). He taught a few people who would eventually reach the level where they could teach others. They would be known as masters. At first, Usui's method was intended to heal people physically, but he later passed on five principles to live by, which he hoped would help people mentally and spiritually.

One of the first Reiki masters, Chujiro Hayashi, divided the training into three levels or "degrees" and introduced a system of payment for Reiki training. He taught Hawayo Takata, who then brought it to America in the 1970s.

Reiki is usually taught to students by a master. Each master will pass on the techniques taught to them, which traces back to the original founder, Mikao Usui. Fortunately, self-Reiki techniques are easy to learn and don't require formal training.

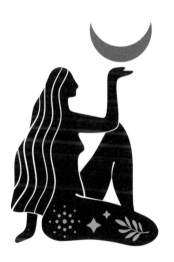

WHAT IS REIKI?

Reiki is a complementary therapy based on the idea that an unseen energy flows through all living things, nourishing and maintaining life.

The word Reiki is made from two Japanese words: rei, which means "all-knowing universal energy", and ki, which means "vital, radiant life energy".

This energy is recognized in many religions and spiritual traditions. It has also been called chi, ki, qi, cosmic energy, prana, the Holy Spirit and life force.

Reiki recognizes the presence of this nourishing flow of energy in all things and aims to direct and use it for positive outcomes. It is mainly done by sending energy into the body, invigorating the body's natural energy flow and clearing any blockages. This is thought to restore harmony and balance in a person's body and emotions.

Reiki is holistic, meaning that it treats the whole person, and its effects can be experienced physically, mentally, emotionally and spiritually. Because Reiki is pure and unconditional, it is open to any belief system and can complement many traditions, cultures and religions, as well as other therapies and modern medicine.

Traditionally, Reiki is taught by master to student. While this is necessary if you wish to treat others professionally, the basic methods are easy to learn and practise by yourself. This book has everything you need to know to be able to practise self-Reiki. Read on and prepare to embrace the life force all around you.

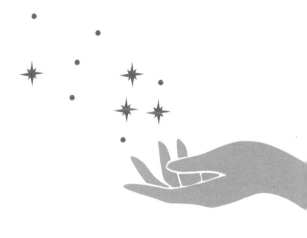

WHERE DOES REIKI ENERGY COME FROM?

It is generally agreed that the source of Reiki energy is a pure and good place of wisdom and love. It has its own intelligence and knows how and where it is needed.

However, nobody truly knows where Reiki energy comes from. There are many ideas and theories, which vary depending on a person's beliefs. People who have a scientific mind look to electromagnetic fields, energy frequencies and even quantum physics. Meanwhile, those seeking a more spiritual source turn to the divine, their god or goddess and angels. Individuals who have a more metaphysical "new age" approach look to the universe, spirit guides and ascended masters, while others think it's pure love.

The beautiful thing about Reiki is that it works for everyone, regardless of their beliefs, nationality, social status, size, colour, religion, sexual orientation, gender or cultural background. It works for the highest good of us all.

You might like to spend some time thinking and researching about what you believe the source of Reiki to be. Or you may be happy to just accept its presence and let it flow. There is no right or wrong approach; it's up to you to decide. What matters is that you are open to it and welcome the healing energy in.

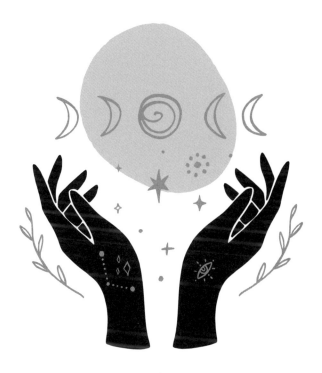

ENERGY FLOW

The constant flow of energy through a human body extends beyond the physical body into one's surroundings (known as an aura). Physical injury, emotional pain and traumatic experiences can create blockages to the natural flow of energy, affecting one's well-being and the body's ability to heal itself.

The practice of Reiki involves consciously opening yourself to the flow of its energy and sending it to where it's needed. This is known as channelling. (See page 61 for more on how to do this.)

Channelling energy into the body realigns and maintains the flow of energy required for well-being and clears blockages. The body can use this to heal itself. Reiki energy is an infinite flow waiting for you to tap into it.

THE GREATEST
FORCE IS THE
DIVINE POWER
WITHIN YOU.

LAILAH GIFTY AKITA

WHAT IS HEALING?

The word "healing" means making something better. People usually think about this in terms of curing physical problems. Reiki works by giving the body a boost of the vital life force energy that nourishes and heals. A Reiki practitioner is the channel through which others can access healing energy, but they are not in control of the outcome – once the energy has passed into another person's body, there is no way of knowing how it will receive and use the energy to heal itself.

Reiki can help ease physical symptoms such as pain and discomfort, and occasionally, there are reports of Reiki miracles totally healing a physical illness. Often, relaxation or a level of acceptance about a physical or emotional problem is needed. Reiki helps because it treats the whole person – body, mind and soul.

Reiki can also be used as a preventative measure, as it helps you to be more relaxed, calm and centred, meaning that you are not as likely to succumb to stress-related conditions, leaving you better equipped to deal with life's ups and downs.

REIKI OUTCOMES

Reiki comes from a place of higher wisdom and perspective. It's intelligent and flows to where it's needed for the best possible outcome, so if you come to Reiki expecting one specific result, you may be surprised to experience results in ways you hadn't considered. For example, you might try Reiki for a back problem aggravated by your job, but it might work by boosting your confidence, leading you to get a different job that's not only better for your back, but that also makes you happier overall. Reiki heals by gently and subtly guiding you, enriching your life by helping you discover new ways of thinking or being and creating a new level of connection with yourself and the world. When practising self-Reiki, try to let go of expectations and be open to however Reiki healing turns up in your life.

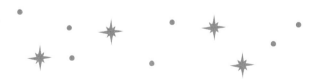

Reiki

works for

the highest

good of all

CHAKRAS AND REIKI

There are seven main chakras in the human body. These are like gateways where energy enters and exits the body. It is important to keep the chakras balanced (the speed of energy flowing at the same rate through each chakra) and keep the energy flowing freely through them to maintain health and a balance of the mind, body and spirit.

Each of the seven main chakras is associated with an area of the body and corresponding physical, mental and emotional states, colours and symbols (explained in the following pages). During Reiki treatment, energy is sent into the body at various positions on or near the chakras. Reiki helps balance out the flow of energy through the chakras, creating harmony throughout. The chakras and the aura (the energy that stretches out beyond the physical body) are known as "the energy body". Reiki treats the whole person: both the physical and energy bodies.

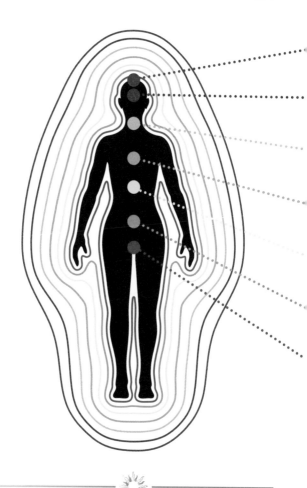

Crown chakra:

Violet, spirituality, "I understand"
Connection with higher self, spirit, source, universe, God or divine wisdom
Linked to the ketheric template layer of aura.

Brow or third eye chakra:

Indigo, awareness, "I see"
Intuition, insight, imagination, intelligence, calm
Linked to the celestial body layer of aura.

Throat chakra:

Blue, communication, "I speak"
Connection, truth, expression, independence
Linked to the etheric template layer of aura.

Heart chakra:

Green, healing, "I love"
Gratitude, compassion for self and others, forgiveness, deep connection
Linked to the astral body layer of aura.

Solar plexus chakra:

Yellow, wisdom, "I do"
Personal power, self-control, vitality, purpose, direction
Linked to mental body layer of aura.

Sacral chakra (hara):

Orange, creativity, "I feel"
Sexuality, feelings, relationships, pleasure, new ideas
Linked to the emotional body layer of aura.

Root chakra:

Red, trust, "I am"
Belonging, safety, self-esteem, connection to the earth
Linked to the etheric body layer of aura.

YOUR AURA EXPLAINED

You have seven auras, each relating to a chakra, colour and condition. Reiki can be given by hovering the hands within the aura, usually in the etheric body layer close to the body.

The etheric layer is associated with the red root chakra. It is the same shape as one's body, sensitive to thoughts and responds well to positive thinking. It includes the physical body, and each successive layer includes the preceding ones.

The emotional body comes next. It is oval shaped and reflects our feelings and emotions. This layer is associated with the orange sacral chakra (*hara*).

The mental body reflects self-knowledge. It is associated with the yellow solar plexus chakra.

The astral body represents unconditional love and is associated with the green heart chakra. It is thought to be the bridge between the physical and spiritual world.

The etheric template is associated with the blue throat chakra. It stores and reflects our memories and thoughts.

The celestial body is linked to the subconscious mind and intuition. It is associated with the indigo third eye (brow) chakra.

The ketheric template is the aura's outer layer. It is connected to the soul and associated with the violet crown chakra.

CHANNELLING ENERGY

Reiki masters reinforce their students' ability to channel Reiki though processes called "attunements" and "empowerments" where certain chakras are opened, and a direct channel to the energy source is created.

When practising self-Reiki, you will channel energy in through the crown chakra on top of your head and out through the chakras on the palms of your hands, into the part of your body where your hands are touching. The hand chakras are in the centre of both palms.

Open your crown chakra by visualizing a lotus flower on the top of your head opening its petals out wide. (See page 46 for more about visualization.)

The sacral chakra, or hara (sometimes also referred to as the *tanden* or *dantien*), is the centre where Reiki energy is stored in the body before it is channelled out again. It is located an inch or two below the navel. (See page 67 for a meditation to familiarize yourself with this chakra.)

BENEFITS OF REIKI

Reiki is inclusive; it's for anyone
who is open to receive it.

Reiki can be used alongside any other
spiritual practice, conventional medicine
or complementary therapy.

Reiki is non-invasive.

Reiki is holistic; it helps the whole person,
physically, mentally and spiritually.

Reiki helps bring comfort, acceptance
and a more positive outlook.

Self-Reiki helps you to feel
empowered to help yourself.

Reiki is intelligent and wise and
flows to where it is needed.

Reiki induces a state of deep relaxation, so
the body is better able to heal itself.

Reiki brings harmony and balance.

Reiki promotes mindfulness.

Reiki helps relieve stress.

Reiki can bring feelings of peace, being
centred and an ability to cope with life.

Reiki relieves pain and discomfort.

ARE THERE ANY SIDE EFFECTS?

Reiki is gentle and non-intrusive, so there are very few side effects. It is normal to feel very relaxed or sleepy after a treatment. Grounding, connecting your body and energy to the earth (see page 54 to learn how to do this) and rest help ease this. Try to enjoy and maintain this relaxed state, as your body heals more effectively when it's relaxed. Many people report sleeping better after a Reiki treatment. You might need to visit the toilet a little more often or sweat more than normal because of the toxins leaving your body. This usually subsides within 24 to 48 hours. Drink plenty of water to rehydrate and assist with detoxification. Try to avoid unhealthy foods, tobacco, alcohol and caffeine after Reiki, as toxins are counterproductive to the body's healing process.

Shifting emotional blockages can result in heightened emotions, so be kind to yourself as these emotions are released. You could start journaling after each session to record anything that you notice over time. You may notice themes and ideas that come up regularly, and it may be helpful to take note of the messages that arise.

THE FIVE PRINCIPLES OF REIKI

- Just for today, I will not worry.
- Just for today, I will not be angry.
- I will honour my parents, teachers and elders.
- I will earn my living honestly.
- I will show gratitude to everything.

The Reiki principles have different meanings for each person, depending on their own values and experiences, so it's a good idea to reflect on what each one means to you. There are several ways to integrate them into your life:

- Repeat them daily
- Meditate on them
- Journal about each one
- Add them to your daily prayers

- Write them out and stick them up where you'll see them regularly

- Set them as a home screen or reminder alert on a phone or device

- Try to live them out in your daily behaviour and actions

The principles are worded with "just for today" to remind you that if you slip up, you can always start again tomorrow. You may wish to check in occasionally to see if your views and ideas around the principles have evolved at all and how embracing them into your life has created positive change.

JUST FOR TODAY, I WILL NOT WORRY

Worry itself is wasteful if it doesn't change anything, and it can lead to anxiety, stress and unhappiness. It can cause an imbalance of the mind, body and spirit and create blockages in the root chakra. Things happen in life that are worrying, but it's how you accept, face, deal with and move on from them that determines your ultimate happiness and well-being. Using tools like self-Reiki, mindfulness and meditation to build your resilience will make you feel better able to cope with whatever comes up.

Putting aside worry and choosing to have a more positive outlook creates a brighter mindset and gives you the best chance at a harmonious, happy life. Remind yourself that you can't predict the future. By spending time worrying about what might never happen, you're stealing your own time and peace of mind.

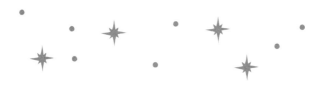

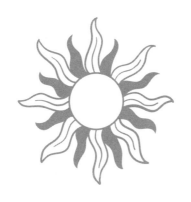

THE GREATEST
MISTAKE YOU CAN
MAKE IN LIFE IS TO
BE CONTINUALLY
FEARING YOU
WILL MAKE ONE.

ELBERT HUBBARD

JUST FOR TODAY, I WILL NOT BE ANGRY

Emotions have a purpose. So, although emotions like anger are seen as negative, it's important to see the message behind them. Channelling the energy of anger into positive action is a constructive way to deal with an often destructive energy. Once anger has served its purpose, it's time to let it go. Be thankful for its presence when you need it and release it. Hanging onto anger long after it has served you can lead to bitterness and create blocks in the flow of energy within you.

While totally eliminating anger from your life may not be realistic, Reiki principles remind you to just focus on one day at a time. Realizing the triggers of your anger and finding ways to react to it that give you back control and free you from old patterns can feel liberating. Read on to discover how self-Reiki can help you find calm and rebalance after you're angry.

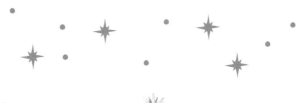

EVERY
MOMENT IS
A FRESH
BEGINNING.

T. S. ELIOT

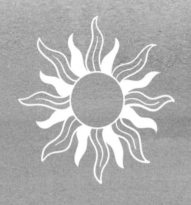

TRY TO BE
A RAINBOW
IN SOMEONE'S
CLOUD.

MAYA ANGELOU

I WILL HONOUR MY PARENTS, TEACHERS, ELDERS AND GUIDES

This principle is often interpreted to be about showing kindness and respect to all living things. Accepting people with differing views and practices can be difficult, but we can use Reiki's limitless love to help us be open and tolerant. Times change, and different generations can have different outlooks on life. But on the whole, people do their best within their means, knowledge and capabilities. Understanding this can help you to accept and respect the actions of your elders and others.

Repeating the principle "I will show kindness and respect to all living things" every day reminds us of the impact of our actions on other living things, including animals and the environment. Try to bring your actions into alignment with your beliefs around this principle. Little drops of kindness and respect create ripples that radiate out, spreading tolerance, love and compassion.

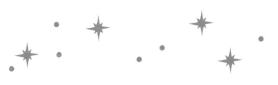

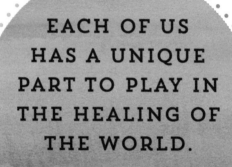

EACH OF US
HAS A UNIQUE
PART TO PLAY IN
THE HEALING OF
THE WORLD.

MARIANNE
WILLIAMSON

I WILL EARN MY LIVING HONESTLY

Earning your living honestly isn't purely about being honest within the work environment or simply finding work that aligns with your beliefs and values. It's also about living out your "soul purpose". This soul work isn't necessarily what brings in the money you need to live on, it could be a hobby or volunteer work; it's what lights you up, something in which you use your natural gifts, express yourself and live out your true calling. Practising self-Reiki and focusing on its principles can support you in living authentically and help you to bring about positive change. Using Reiki to increase self-awareness and emotional well-being creates a clear flow of energy through you, making it easier for you to manifest the life you want and deserve. When your energy is aligned with your desires, it's easier to live your truth.

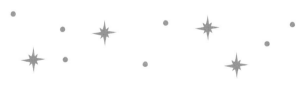

I WILL SHOW GRATITUDE TO EVERYTHING

Taking a moment to appreciate all of the good things in your life really helps to lift your spirits. There is joy to be found in so many things: loved ones, health, being outdoors, clear blue skies, trees, birdsong, street performers, sunsets, laughter – the list is endless. Finding value and gratitude for these blessings helps you to put more materialistic things and your pursuit of them (which is often exhausting and fraught with stress) in perspective.

Being mindfully grateful helps you find the good in any situation, which, in turn, reduces the chances of anger and bitterness taking hold. Gratitude puts you in a positive state of mind, which attracts more blessings. Create a daily practice of listing three things you are grateful for. This simple exercise can really improve your sense of well-being. Having gratitude for Reiki will also help strengthen your connection to its source and helps you be a clear channel.

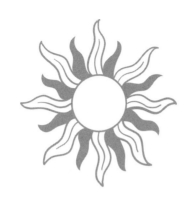

THERE IS ALWAYS
SOMETHING TO BE
GRATEFUL FOR.

RHONDA BYRNE

You are

safe, you

are loved

PRACTISING REIKI

Regular Reiki treatments are great for maintaining your health and well-being. You can either book treatments with a Reiki practitioner or try self-Reiki. You might find that using self-Reiki gives you a boost between visits to your practitioner.

Self-Reiki can be carried out as often as you feel necessary and whenever suits you. You might like to do it first thing in the morning before you get out of bed, add it to the relaxation or warm down part of physical exercise, include it in any meditation, prayer or other spiritual practices you already have or make time for it at bedtime as a way to relax before sleeping.

The following chapter will teach you everything you need to begin the beautiful practice of self-Reiki. You will find instructions, exercises and tips which will often tell you to hold a position or practise an exercise for as long as you wish or to tweak an idea to suit you. This puts the power in your hands (literally!). Experiment, trust your experiences and learn to judge for yourself what serves you best. Building your Reiki practice in your own way makes your personal connection to it all the stronger. Trust yourself and trust Reiki.

WHAT TO EXPECT

A Reiki practitioner should welcome you and make you feel comfortable and relaxed. They will start by asking you a few questions about your health and lifestyle to help them understand your needs and become aware of any health issues that might affect the treatment. You will remain clothed and lie down or sit in a relaxed position while the practitioner places their hands in a series of nonintrusive positions on or near your body. Treatments tend to last 30 minutes to an hour.

Reiki practitioners are not trained in diagnosis and will not predict any specific outcome from treatment. You may or may not feel sensations during treatment. Some of the most common sensations include deep relaxation, sleep, heat, tingling and seeing lights and colours. Sometimes, releasing an energy blockage can cause you to cry. This is perfectly normal; allow the emotions to flow and let them pass. Afterward, most people feel calm with a peaceful sense of well-being on all levels.

YOUR

INNER LIGHT

SHINES

BRIGHTLY

REIKI TOUCH

Touch has the power to comfort, reassure and create bonds. How often do people hug their loved ones, give a comforting squeeze to someone's arm, shake hands or high five without thinking about why they're doing it? When you're hurt, your instinct is to rub the pain away. Humans instinctively understand the positive power of touch, and channelling Reiki into the touch enhances its benefits.

Not everyone feels comfortable with the "hands-on" element of visiting a Reiki practitioner. But Reiki works just as well with the practitioner's hands hovering near the body but not touching it. A good Reiki practitioner will be willing and open to having a conversation with you about what you feel comfortable with. It's okay at any point during a Reiki treatment to ask the practitioner to stop or move their hands.

During self-Reiki, you might find issues about touching yourself come up, but it's likely that Reiki will help you process these and find a new level of comfort with your own body. Let your intuition guide you.

HOW TO PRACTISE SELF-REIKI

In this chapter, you will discover how the power of your mind influences the flow of energy using intention and visualization, the hand positions and the simple but powerful techniques required for self-Reiki.

SETTING AN INTENTION

Your intention is your aim or purpose. It influences the flow and effectiveness of Reiki energy. Thinking of the aims and outcomes you hope for while channelling Reiki energy tells the energy where to go and how it should work. You might have a very specific intention like easing a headache, mending a pulled muscle or calming anxiety. Or your intention might be more general and be about something like relaxation or improving your well-being. Hold your intention in your mind while channelling Reiki energy to direct it to where you want it. Try to keep your intentions simple and clear. For example, "I'm using Reiki to get rid of this headache." This is easy for the Reiki energy to follow and also helps you to assess how well it is working. Just having the intention that Reiki will work for the highest good is often the best option.

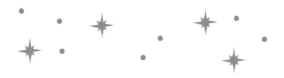

TRY,
REALLY TRY.
THINK,
REALLY THINK.
BELIEVE,
REALLY BELIEVE.

NORMAN VINCENT
PEALE

LEARN TO VISUALIZE

One of the most useful techniques in Reiki is visualization, which is using your imagination to create an image in your mind. This is a powerful way to influence your physical and energetic body and the flow of Reiki energy. Some people find it easier than others to "see" pictures in their minds. Practice helps to build this skill.

You can use the power of visualizations to direct the flow of energy by "seeing" it flow where you want it to and open and close your chakras by visualizing it happening. You may visualize Reiki energy in different ways: as a white beam of light, a silvery fluid or a golden thread. Chakras can often look like flowers with open petals or spinning funnels.

There is no right or wrong way to imagine them, and visualizations will not look the same for everyone. Visualizing is going to work better if those images feel real and true to you, rather than guessing what something "should" look like.

If you find it hard to visualize images in your mind, don't worry. Intention is the most important part. Just keep your intention clear in your mind by repeating it to yourself and believe that it will happen.

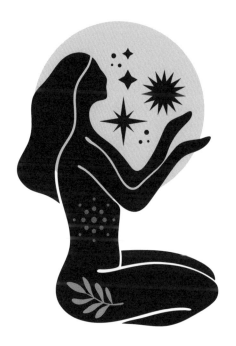

A VISUALIZATION EXERCISE

Here's a simple exercise to experience the power of visualization:

You are going to visualize a lemon. In your mind, see its dimpled, shiny, yellow skin. Think about how it would feel to touch. Really study the lemon in as much detail as you can. Picture yourself pushing a fingernail into the skin, breaking the surface and exposing the pale pith. Next, see yourself bringing the lemon to your nose and inhaling. What would it smell like? Now, visualize cutting into the lemon, the juice bursting out and covering your fingers. Lastly, bite into the lemon and suck the juice.

How did your mind build this picture for you? Did your body react by making your mouth water?

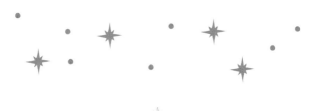

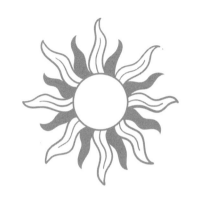

IMAGINATION IS
THE BEGINNING
OF CREATION.

GEORGE BERNARD SHAW

TRUST YOUR INTUITION

Your intuition is your inner sense of truth that you just know is correct without having proof. It's not called your gut feeling for nothing; it's often felt physically in the stomach or abdomen. Learn to listen to this inner voice and see what happens when you trust its guidance. Often in Reiki, you will be called on to trust your intuition, and this gets easier with practice. For example, you'll need to use your intuition to know how long to hold each hand position. Try not to question or second guess yourself. Just go with what feels right and trust Reiki to guide you. Remember that Reiki only works for the highest good and can do no harm, so you can't really go wrong with it.

Power and

potential are

within you

CREATE A SANCTUARY

The first thing to do when practicing self-Reiki is to create a quiet space for yourself. You will need somewhere to lie down or recline comfortably, so you might want to gather some cushions and blankets. Make sure the temperature is comfortable and that your space is inviting. You might like to include relaxing music, dimmed lights, pleasant scents and textures or whatever you need to feel safe and at ease.

Decide how long you want to make your self-Reiki session and add it to your schedule to make sure it happens. Tell others you can't be reached during this time so that you will not be interrupted. Lock your door, put up a "do not disturb" sign and switch your phone off. This is the time to focus on you.

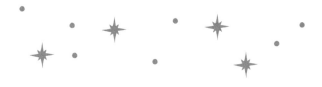

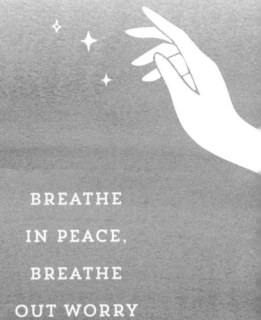

BREATHE
IN PEACE,
BREATHE
OUT WORRY

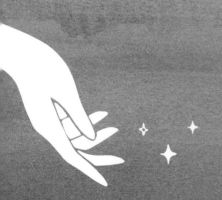

GROUNDING

Grounding means connecting your body and energy to the earth. Creating this connection helps you to be mindfully present in your physical body and in the moment. It brings your awareness within, helping you to concentrate on the here and now. Your connection to the earth enables you to absorb its energy and also provides an escape route for excess energy during Reiki treatments. Take a moment to ground yourself before and after each self-Reiki treatment, meditation or exercise, as it tends to make you more present, mindful and calm and can help to alleviate anxiety and panic.

You can ground yourself simply by focusing on where your body connects to the earth – your feet if you are standing, bottom if you are sitting and back if you are lying down. Feel the physical pressure and contact between you and your point of contact with the earth (this could be the floor, a seat, bed or, better still, the ground outside) and see if you can sense an energetic connection too.

Other grounding techniques:

- Focus on the soles of your feet
- Massage your feet or hands
- Stamp your feet
- Drink water
- Stretch your body
- Dance
- Take a shower or bath
- Take a walk
- Lay on the ground
- Walk barefoot
- Put your hands in the soil
- Hug a tree

Pay attention to your senses; focus on what you can see, hear, touch, taste and smell. Use whichever method works for you, depending on the time and suitability.

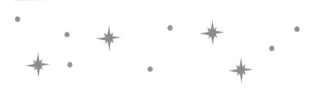

A GROUNDING MEDITATION

1   Sit or stand with your feet flat on the floor.

2   Visualize roots growing from the bottom of your feet, making their way down into the earth.

3   See your roots going deeper into the earth, wrapping around rocks and tree roots, and anchoring you much like a tree.

4   Allow these roots to go so deep that they reach the centre of the earth, where you see a huge crystal. Visualize your roots wrapping around the crystal connecting you there. Intend that the earth's energy travels up your roots like water does with tree roots. Visualize the energy coming all the way up from the centre of the earth and into your body.

5   Take time to feel the earth's energy and how it affects you. At first, you might not notice anything, but with time, you might detect a buzzing or fizzing sensation in your feet that travels up your legs as the energy rises within you. You may feel a sense of gravity

pulling you to the earth, a real awareness of being in your physical body, or a deep sense of calm or a mindful awareness of being in the present moment.

6 Continue this visualization as long as you wish. Then send thoughts of love and gratitude down your roots into the earth in return for its energy.

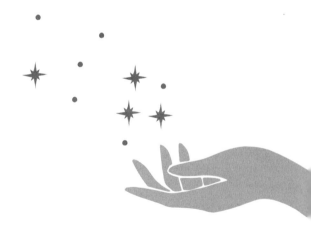

SWITCH ON REIKI

Some people like to have a specific action or set of words that they say in order to "switch on" or start the flow of Reiki before they begin to treat someone or do self-Reiki. This could be rubbing their hands together, placing their hands in *gassho* (prayer position) or saying words like "Reiki on" or repeating "Reiki, Reiki, Reiki."

You might like to include gratitude for Reiki or invoke a feeling of unconditional love as you switch on Reiki. Keep it as simple as you can in order to stay focused on your connection to the Reiki source and not be distracted by complicated words or actions. Experiment with what works for you by trying each method a few times and seeing how they affect the way Reiki begins to flow for you, and how you feel during and after the self-Reiki.

Once you have found a way to switch on the Reiki flow that works for you, use this each time you begin to channel it. Remember that as your relationship with Reiki grows, your methods may change, and you might find you need to switch to a different method. Sometimes, just thinking about Reiki can start the flow, and some people find that Reiki starts flowing spontaneously when they need it. Reiki is a unique experience for each person. Trust yourself to decide what works for you.

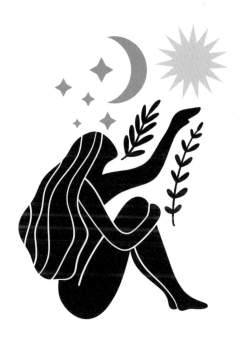

Be true
to yourself.
Forgive yourself.
Love yourself.

PREPARING FOR SELF-REIKI

First, visualize your crown chakra (top of your head) opening to receive Reiki energy. Have the intention that you are open and ready for channelling.

Now, ask Reiki to allow you to channel the energy into yourself and state in your mind or out loud that you will receive Reiki for the highest good of all.

Visualize the energy (often seen as a pure white light) entering your crown chakra from above and flowing into your body, filling you with light. You might be able to feel it gathering in your hara/sacral chakra as a tingling or warm sensation.

Next, place your hands together, rub them a little to feel the energy in your palms and then settle them into a prayer position. Have the intention that the energy is flowing out of them. To help with this, use visualization and any words that "switch on" Reiki for you.

You might feel a warm or tingling sensation or a sense of pressure pushing your hands apart. If you can't feel anything, don't worry. Just trust that Reiki works and keep going.

You are now channelling Reiki energy into your body through your crown chakra and out through your palm chakras. Try slowly moving your hands closer together and further apart to see if you can sense the energy between them. Don't try to force the flow. Just allow it to happen. Do this for as long as you need to familiarize yourself with the energy. When you feel ready, you can move your hands to the first hand position (see page 64).

You are now ready to give yourself Reiki.

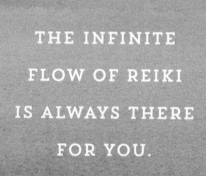

THE INFINITE
FLOW OF REIKI
IS ALWAYS THERE
FOR YOU.

HAND POSITIONS

First: Eyes

Place your hands over your face, gently
cupping your eyes and resting your
fingers on your forehead. This treats
the eyes, third eye/brow chakra,
pituitary gland and sinuses. It helps
you recover from colds, eases
stress and aids intuition.

Second: Crown Chakra

Place your hands either side your head,
with your fingers meeting over the
crown chakra. This treats the crown
chakra and the pineal gland,
balances the left and right
side of the brain and helps
with headaches, depression,
memory and mental clarity.

Third: Sides of the Head

Place your hands over your ears. This treats the ears, pineal gland and thyroid. It helps with balance and hearing, eases earaches and brings comfort to the whole body.

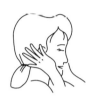

Fourth: Back of the Head

Place your hands behind and underneath your head. This treats the back of the brain and brow chakra. It helps improve coordination, treats headaches and insomnia, aids relaxation and induces a feeling of security, relieving fears.

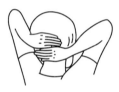

Fifth: Brow Chakra

Place one hand on your forehead and one behind your head. This clears and opens the brow chakra ("third eye"), opening your intuition and helps with tension headaches and upset emotions. It is also useful for treating exhaustion.

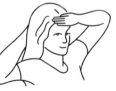

Sixth: Throat

Place your hands around your throat, with your wrists touching together. This treats the neck, thyroid gland and throat chakra. It also helps the lymphatic system, a sore throat, vocal cords and self-expression.

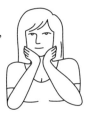

Seventh: Heart and Thymus

Place one hand over your heart (the centre of your chest between your nipples) and one just above it over the thymus gland (central upper chest). This treats the thymus/immune system, heart, lungs and heart chakra, helping with breathing and emotional problems.

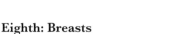

Eighth: Breasts

Place one hand on each breast. This treats the lungs and breasts and aids the flow of lymph in this area.

Ninth: Solar Plexus

Place your hands on your lower rib cage below the sternum on each side of your body or place one hand over the other in this area. This treats the solar plexus chakra and stomach.

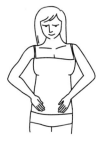

It helps reduce fear and anger and promotes calmness.

Tenth: Sacral Chakra

Place hands on the sacral chakra (or hara) just below your navel. This treats the lower organs and sacral chakra. It is calming for the nerves and stress, as well as aiding your metabolism and calming powerful emotions. Placing one hand on the hara and one on the brow balances the body and creates a sense of calmness.

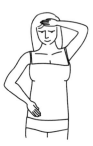

Eleventh: Pelvis

Place your hands over your lower abdomen/groin. This treats the large intestine, reproductive organs, bladder, hips and root chakra. It also helps with menstrual problems and PMS and also helps to release guilt.

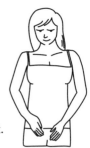

Twelfth: Kidneys

Place your hands either side of your back, over your kidneys. This treats the kidneys, adrenal glands and the middle of your back and helps to build energy. It is good for detoxing, relieving back pain and boosting self-confidence.

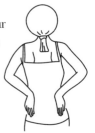

Thirteenth: Sacrum

Place your hands under your lower back, covering the sacrum (bottom of the spine). This treats your lower back, hips and root chakra.

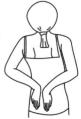

Fourteenth: Hug

Wrap your arms around your body, placing your hands on your ribs or shoulders. Give yourself a hug and send yourself unconditional love. This treats the chest and upper body area and also works on self-acceptance and self-love.

Any positions that are difficult for you can be adapted to suit your mobility. Place your hands as close as you comfortably can and send the Reiki energy to the spot you need it using intention and visualization. You are not limited to the hand positions described here. Follow your intuition and place your hands wherever you feel guided to.

LET IT FLOW

Let the Reiki energy flow from your hands into your body at each hand position (see page 64). Hold each position for as long as you feel necessary. You may feel warmth, tingling, a static sensation, fizzing or bubbling where your hands are in contact with your body, or you may not notice anything at all. Hold each position for about 3–5 minutes, or longer if you feel you need it. You may notice the sensations slow or stop when you need to move to the next hand position, or just feel that it's time. With practice, you will learn to trust your instincts as to how long to stay in each hand position.

When switching between hand positions, it is gentler to move one hand at a time so that there is always one hand in contact with your body. This means there is a more constant flow of energy.

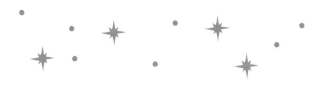

WHAT
DRAINS YOUR
SPIRIT DRAINS
YOUR BODY.
WHAT FUELS YOUR
SPIRIT FUELS
YOUR BODY.

CAROLINE MYSS

Let go,
let flow

REIKI AND MEDITATION

Meditation is a popular practice in which you train your mind to focus on one thing in order to create mental clarity and emotional calm. The good news is that Reiki can be easily combined with meditation – simply switch on Reiki while meditating!

Reiki's healing effects will help calm your mind and boost meditation. The Reiki meditations throughout this book do not require you to clear your mind, which can often seem too difficult. Instead, they will ask you to focus on a visualization or intention, helping to keep obtrusive thoughts out. However, if you do find your mind wandering or unwanted thoughts popping in, don't stress about it. Simply bring your attention back to the meditation and carry on. If you are new to meditating, try one every few days and don't focus for too long to begin with. Don't forget to begin and end your meditations with grounding (see page 54). Read on to learn a simple Reiki meditation.

A SIMPLE REIKI MEDITATION

This meditation will help familiarize you with the sensations of Reiki and your hara/sacral chakra.

1   Sit or lie comfortably, close your eyes and take three deep breaths.

2   Focus on your hara, the sacral chakra (below your navel). This is the energy centre in which Reiki is stored when it enters the body. Visualize it bathed in an orange glow.

3   Switch on Reiki and imagine the Reiki energy flowing in as you inhale.

4   Let the Reiki energy flow in when you breathe in and pour into your hara.

5   In the pause before you exhale, focus on your hara and how it feels with the energy there.

6   Exhale and visualize the energy leaving your hara, flowing out of you in all directions as you breathe out.

7   Repeat steps 4, 5 and 6 while maintaining the focus on your hara and the energy flowing in and out of it.

REIKI BUBBLE

Reiki bubbles are most often used for love and/or protection. You can place yourself in a Reiki bubble anytime and anywhere with this simple technique:

1 Take a few slow, calm breaths.

2 Begin to channel Reiki in the way that works best for you.

3 Visualize Reiki energy entering your crown chakra and filling your body.

4 Once you feel your body is full of energy, allow it to flow out of you in all directions, filling your aura and the space around you.

5 Allow this bubble of Reiki energy to stretch out beyond your arms, reach to whatever size feels comfortable to you.

6 Intend for the surface of this bubble to be strong, one that can only be penetrated by love and positivity. Go about your day knowing that you are held safe and protected inside your Reiki bubble, surrounded by love.

REIKI BALL

This exercise shows how to create a ball of Reiki energy between your hands. It's a good way to familiarize yourself with the sensations of channelling Reiki.

1   Place your hands into the prayer position, with your palms together in front of you.

2   Say "Reiki on" or start channelling Reiki in any way that works for you.

3   Sense the energy building between your hands. Does it feel heavy, fizzy or light and bubbly? There is no wrong way to sense energy, just what feels right to you. You might begin to feel the pressure of the energy pushing your hands apart. Gradually separate your hands and hold the energy between them. You might like to cup your hands at this point to hold the ball of energy that is forming.

4   Try pulling your hands further apart and then pressing them back together and see if this changes the way the energy feels. Familiarize yourself with the sensations and experiment.

5 Once you have finished with the Reiki ball, you can give it to yourself by moving your hands to your body and "tipping" the energy into your heart chakra or over your head into your crown chakra. Alternatively, you can give the energy to the universe by opening your hands and letting it go or send it into the earth by placing the ball on the ground.

6 Feel gratitude for the energy you have been using.

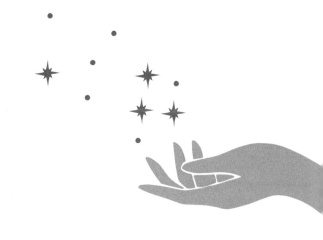

TAP INTO THE SOURCE

As we discussed earlier in the book (page 12), nobody truly knows the source of Reiki energy, but it's agreed that it comes from a place of wisdom, and its love is pure and good. How you choose to view the source of Reiki energy is up to you and often depends on your beliefs. Here's how to meditate on what it means to you and strengthen your connection.

1   Sit or lie comfortably, close your eyes and take three deep breaths.

2   Visualize roots, pipes or a chain or rope growing from the part of you that is touching or closest to the ground, into the earth, connecting at its core (this will be your feet if you are sitting or base of the spine if lying down). Know this connects you to the centre of the earth and that you are grounded and safe.

3   Bring your awareness to the crown chakra (top of head) and picture a flower there opening its petals wide to receive the energy.

4   Switch on Reiki and allow the energy to flow into your crown chakra.

5   Visualize a strong cord, rope or pipe growing out of your crown chakra/flower, going up and up, into the infinite space and connecting to the source – whatever you believe that to be.

6   Continue this meditation for as long as you wish.

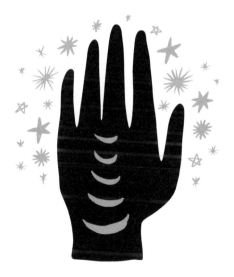

STRENGTHEN YOUR REIKI ENERGY

This exercise, called Hatsu Rei Ho, is a series of short meditations intended to "start up" or strengthen the flow of Reiki energy. It makes a beautiful daily practice that strengthens and maintains your connection to Reiki and helps you to live out the key principles.

Follow the steps below. At first, you will need to look at these pages to remind and guide you, but with regular practice, Hatsu Rei Ho becomes second nature.

Step One: Relax

Sit in a relaxed position with your hands in your lap. Take your focus to your *hara* (sacral chakra) about two inches below your navel and close your eyes.

Step Two: Focus

State your intention. Try something simple like "I am now going to do Hatsu Rei Ho" or "I am connecting to Reiki."

Step Three: Brushing Off

This technique cleanses your aura, brushing off stagnant energy.

1   Place your right hand flat on the left side of your chest, with your fingers pointing to your shoulder. Exhale as you sweep your hand diagonally across your body and over your chest, passing over the sternum and finishing at the right hip.

2   Repeat this with your left hand beginning at the right side of your chest and finishing at the left hip, exhaling as you go. Repeat this again with your right hand starting on the left side.

3   Stretch out your left arm in front of you with your palm facing downward. Keep your left arm in this position while you place your right hand on your shoulder. Exhale as you sweep it down your left arm, brushing right off the end of your fingertips.

4   Repeat the same action, brushing your left hand down your right arm and then again on the left side. Remember to exhale as you do this. If it helps, you can visualize brushing away stagnant energy from your aura.

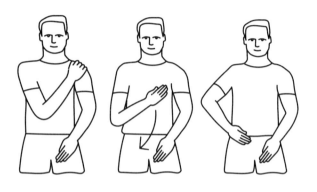

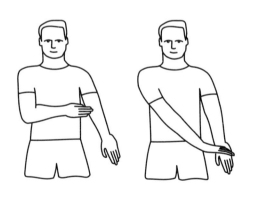

Step Four: Connect to Reiki

Stretch your arms up above your head, palms upward, and your fingers facing inward to each other. Connect to Reiki. Visualize and feel the energy flowing into your hands, down your arms and into your body.

Once you feel the flow of energy, lower your hands gently back into your lap with your palms upward.

Step Five: Purify the Spirit

This is a technique known as "the cleansing breath".

1   Stay in a relaxed pose with your palms upward in your lap and focus on your hara again. Inhale and visualize the energy pouring into your crown chakra, through your body and into your hara. Take a pause before you exhale as you feel the energy spreading throughout your body.

2   Exhale, visualizing the energy radiating out of your body in all directions into infinity. Repeat these breaths while visualizing the flow of energy into you, filling you and flowing out of you. Do this for a couple of minutes or longer if you'd like. You may start to notice the energy tingling in the palms of your hands.

Step Six: *Gassho*

Place your hands together in a prayer position, with your palms together in front of your chest, slightly higher than your heart. If you are in the correct position, you should be able to breathe onto your fingertips. Take your attention to the point where your two middle fingers are touching.

Step Seven: Breathing

1   Keep your hands in the *gassho* position and breathe in deeply.

2   As you inhale, visualize Reiki energy entering your hands and flowing down your arms into your *hara*.

3   As you exhale, allow the energy to flow back up your arms and out of your hands. Do this for a few minutes or longer.

Step Eight: The Reiki Principles

Repeat the Reiki principles aloud three times and contemplate what each of them means to you:
Just for today, I will not worry.
Just for today, I will not be angry.

I will honour my parents, teachers, elders and guides.
I will earn my living honestly.
I will show gratitude to everything.

Step Nine: Focus

Place your palms down in your lap. Open your eyes and say to yourself: "I have finished Hatsu Rei Ho." Shake your hands and stamp your feet a little to ground yourself again.

> Spend as long as you like at steps 4, 5, 6 and 7. Some days, you might have more time, but daily repetition can become the basis for a meaningful spiritual practice that will enrich your life.

REIKI FOR SLEEP

Self-Reiki is deeply relaxing, so it's no surprise that it can help with insomnia. It can calm your racing thoughts, allowing you to drift into a peaceful, restorative sleep.

Here's how to add Reiki to your bedtime regimen:

1 Get into your normal, comfortable sleeping position.

2 Place one hand on your brow chakra (forehead) and the other on your solar plexus (stomach).

3 Switch on Reiki with the intention of relaxation and sleep.

4 Take three to five deep, slow breaths.

5 Notice your stomach rising and falling each time you breathe in and out.

6 Return your breathing to a normal pace and continue self-Reiki in this position for about 10 minutes or as long as it takes to feel deeply relaxed.

7 Maintain this relaxed state and slowly remove your hands, or continue self-Reiki until you fall asleep.

REIKI FOR CREATIVITY

Creativity is a wonderful way to be mindful, allowing you to be present in the moment, as well as calming your mind and body. And if you switch on Reiki while you create, you will charge both yourself and your creations with Reiki energy. There are many ways to be creative besides art and crafts: cooking and baking, dancing, singing, writing, journaling, arranging displays of natural objects, decorating your home, scrapbooking, photography, arranging furniture and objects in your home, mixing essential oils, putting together gift hampers... the list could go on. All of these activities can be done while channelling Reiki. Here's how...

Switch on Reiki so that the energy is flowing in through your crown chakra and out through your hands. Begin your creative task with the intention that the energy is channelled into whatever you are making. Regardless of whether it's a photograph, ornament display or a doodle, it will be charged with Reiki and radiate its energy.

EMERGENCY REIKI

Planning and creating a sumptuous space for a luxurious self-Reiki treatment is wonderful, but there are times when you need emergency treatment. Sometimes, things happen during your day that a little bit of self-Reiki could help. This could be an emotional issue like a moment of discomfort or nervousness about a difficult conversation you are about to have. Or it could be a physical issue like a scratch or pulled muscle.

Firstly, make sure you are safe and away from any immediate physical danger and move away from any emotional triggers if possible. Once you are physically safe, you can start to channel Reiki and use it however best suits the situation. Here are some suggestions:

- Visualize yourself surrounded by a Reiki bubble of love and protection (see page 75 for how to do this).

- Place your hands on or near a wound and channel Reiki into the area.

- Channel Reiki out of your hands into the room with the intention of creating a calm, peaceful atmosphere.

- Place your hands on your throat and channel Reiki into your throat chakra to help with communication.

- Place your hands on your heart chakra and channel Reiki into your heart to heal emotional pain.

- Visualize Reiki energy coming in through your nose when you inhale and anxiety coming out of your mouth when you exhale. Take some slow, deep breaths and feel the calming influence of Reiki.

- Just say "Reiki", either out loud or in your mind, and trust it to flow to where it is needed.

You are not limited to these suggestions. Reiki is intelligent and will guide you to the best way to use it. Trust your instincts and Reiki.

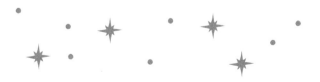

REIKI FOR SPECIFIC BODY PAIN

Humans instinctively place their hand over a painful area or rub where it hurts, so you probably already automatically do this for specific body pain. To add the healing benefits of Reiki, channel energy out of your hands (as described on page 61).

Place your hands over the affected area or hover them just above if it hurts to touch and channel Reiki into the area while intending to ease the pain. Depending on the size of the painful area, you may need to move your hands to new positions until all of the area has been treated. If the painful spot is out of reach or if pain limits your movement, you can place your hand as near as possible to the pain and send the Reiki energy to the area by visualizing it flowing there and holding the intention that it flows to where it is needed. For example, for back pain, place your hand on the front of your body and send the Reiki through your body to your back. If you can't move at all, just begin to channel Reiki, ask it to go to where it is needed and visualize the pure light energy filling this area.

You can vary the treatments depending on the situation and cause of your pain. A stubbed toe may only require a few minutes as a one-off "emergency" treatment; chronic pain or a long-term injury may require at least one longer treatment a day. Experiment to see what works for you. Start with 5 or 10 minutes of self-Reiki on the painful area and increase the length or frequency as needed. Quite often, people find that even if the pain doesn't completely disappear, Reiki gives them some relief, helps them find acceptance and makes them feel empowered to cope.

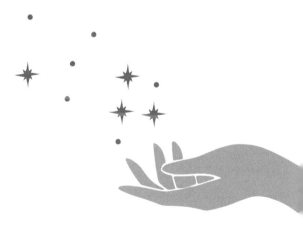

REIKI FOR ANXIETY

Regular Reiki treatments help maintain well-being, resilience, positivity and calmness. After using Reiki for a while, you might find yourself less anxious. When you do feel anxiety rising use one or a combination of these quick Reiki hand positions and tips to help you regain control.

Take five slow breaths, inhaling calming Reiki energy and exhaling anxiety.

Place your hands on your ribs, feel them move with your breaths and channel Reiki there for a few minutes.

Channel Reiki into Your Head

This can be done different ways depending on your location. If you are sitting at a desk, you might want to discreetly place your hands on your temples, forehead or behind your head. Another subtle position is resting your chin in your hand, visualizing Reiki energy flowing into your head. Place your hands over your eyes in the first hand position (see page 64) to make yourself calm. If you can, lie down on your back with your hands behind your head, cradling the weight of your head (literally taking the weight off your mind) and channel Reiki in this position for a few minutes.

Repeat the Reiki principles to yourself three times. This will help you pause and gain a new perspective, reminding you not to worry and that each day is a new start.

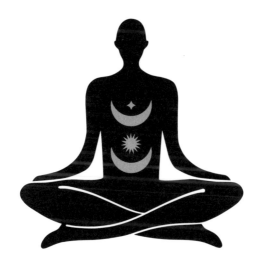

A MEDITATION FOR BELONGING

This meditation helps you feel a sense of belonging, both on the planet and in this moment.

1   Sit comfortably with your feet flat on the ground, close your eyes and take three deep breaths.

2   Ground yourself by connecting to the earth however you like. Know that you are connected to the centre of the earth and that you are grounded and safe.

3   Visualize earth energy flowing up into your feet, up your legs and filling your body.

4   Open your crown chakra by visualizing it unfolding like a flower.

5   Switch on Reiki and allow it to flow into your crown chakra. Imagine it filling your body.

6   Feel or picture the earth and Reiki energy combining and spreading throughout your body.

7   As you exhale, visualize yourself sending the combined energy out of your feet into the earth and

out of your crown chakra to whatever you personally believe the source of Reiki energy to be.

8   Know that you belong in this space and in this moment, connected to both the earth and source. No one else can fill this space but you. You are vital, important and needed.

9   At this point, you can send thoughts of love, peace and gratitude with the energy to the earth and source.

Continue this meditation for as long as you wish.

Your footprints
mark your place
on the earth.

Wherever they
are, that's
where you belong.

ENJOY A REIKI BATH

Give yourself a glorious self-Reiki treatment with the added benefits of a beautiful, warm bath. Do this for yourself and make sure you will not be disturbed. You can make this a nourishing experience by including any of the following:

- Add essential oils, bath salts, herbs or flowers of your choice
- Play relaxing music
- Place candles around the bath
- Dim the lights
- Place crystals near the bath

Once you are comfortable in the bath, place your hands in a prayer position and begin to channel Reiki. Starting at your crown chakra, work through the hand positions and channel Reiki for a few minutes at each position, just as you would in a normal self-Reiki treatment. To enhance the holistic experience of Reiki, don't forget to repeat the Reiki principles to yourself as well.

TRY A REIKI SHOWER

Just like the Reiki bath, you can enhance your shower with Reiki too. In your shower, switch on Reiki and visualize energy flowing from above with the water. Stand under the water, letting it fall on your crown chakra. Let it flow over you and know that Reiki is also flowing over and through you, cleansing you inside and out, removing blocks and stagnant energy as it goes.

You can also perform a Reiki shower without water. Switch on Reiki and stretch your arms over your head, with your palms down. Visualize the Reiki energy as it showers down on you, sweeping away negativity and leaving you feeling revitalized.

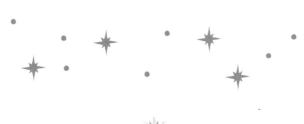

YOU ARE

ABUNDANT

WITH HEALTH,

LOVE AND

JOY

DRINK REIKI WATER

Reiki can be used to charge and bless your drinking water. Hold a glass of water in your hands or place a hand over it. Begin to channel Reiki and send the energy out of your hands into the water with the intention of charging or blessing it with positive energy. You can just be generally positive with this or have a specific intention. Some examples of intentions for drinking water would be that the water will cleanse and detox you or help calm an upset stomach.

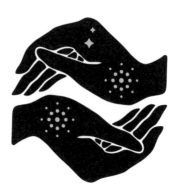

CHANNEL REIKI INTO YOUR FOOD

You can use Reiki to charge and bless your food like with water. Simply place your hands above the cooking pan at a safe height, taking care not to burn yourself on any hot steam, or wait for the food to be on the plate when serving. Then channel Reiki energy into the food to charge and bless it. You can hold the intention of filling your food with general positivity or you can be more specific and intend that it is nourishing and tasty for example.

Don't forget the Reiki principle about gratitude. While using Reiki on your food and water, take a moment to be grateful for the whole process that brought it to you. Think about the incredible water cycle that nature provides and the ingenious way humans use it to provide you with clean drinking water. Consider the forces of nature, sun and rain, fertile soil and humans working in harmony to grow your food. Be grateful for everything that went into getting the food to you and remember all the people involved – including yourself!

REIKI FOR THE ENVIRONMENT

Eco-anxiety (anxiety about environmental and ecological damage) is common, but you can feel empowered to make a positive impact by using Reiki to benefit the parts of your environment that are within your reach. Read on to find out how.

Reiki for Plants – Plants flourish when they receive positivity. Along with talking nicely to your house or garden plants, channel Reiki energy into them. Hold your hands near them and send them Reiki with intentions for growth and health. You can channel Reiki energy to fruit and vegetable plants with the intention they yield a good harvest full of goodness and flavour. Any surplus energy will go into the earth.

Reiki for Your Pets – Switch on Reiki and see how your pet reacts to you stroking them while channelling Reiki out of your hands.

Reiki for Trees – Place your palms on the tree and channel Reiki out of your hands into it. Focus on gratitude for its strength and the work it does to purify the air. Use the opportunity to ground yourself by taking your attention to the tree's roots; visualize roots growing from your feet and into the ground entwining with the tree roots and anchoring you to the earth.

Reiki for Your Rubbish – This sounds like a weird idea, but a lot of rubbish gets sent into the earth in landfill sites. If you hold your hands over your rubbish bags and channel Reiki into them before they get taken away, at least you can send them into the earth with Reiki energy and positive intentions of healing for the planet.

Reiki for the Earth – Place your hands on the ground and channel Reiki into the earth. Visualize it going deep into the planet and being used for healing and correcting environmental imbalances. You can do this while also grounding; there's a lovely balance between receiving energy from the earth and sending energy back into it that reminds you that you are just where you belong.

MEDITATION FOR THE WORLD AND BEYOND

This meditation instils a sense of connection to the wider world. It enables you to send Reiki energy out with intention of bringing its healing to the world and out into the universe/source of Reiki/anything else you believe in.

1   Sit or lie comfortably, close your eyes and take three deep breaths.

2   Ground yourself by connecting to the earth in whichever way suits you. Know that you are connected to the centre of the earth and that you are grounded and safe.

3   Breathe Reiki into your hara as you inhale and out again as you exhale, as described in steps 4, 5 and 6 of the simple meditation on page 74.

4   Once you feel comfortable doing this for a few breaths, bring your attention to the energy radiating out of you as you exhale, sending it out further each time you breathe out.

5   Visualize the Reiki energy as a pure light flowing out so far it fills your room.

6   Next, send the energy out to fill the whole building – if you are outdoors, adapt this to the field, forest or wherever you are.

7   When you next exhale, the energy floods out of the building to your surrounding area.

8   Continue to send the energy further with each exhalation. Try to flood your town with its light and, eventually, country.

9   As the energy stretches out further, take a wider perspective with your visualization. See the light from a point above the earth and see it spreading across the land and oceans, eventually wrapping around the world.

10 Send the energy in all directions out into the universe. You can also send out thoughts of healing, love and peace to all creation and gratitude to the source of it all (whatever you believe that to be).

11 Slowly bring the energy back to the world, across the countries to your area, your building, your room and finally back into yourself.

12 Take your awareness back to your connection to the earth and feel grounded and safe.

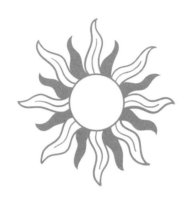

DON'T WASTE
THE EARTH –
IT IS OUR
JEWEL.

BUZZ ALDRIN

REIKI FOR YOUR SPACE

Reiki can be used to improve the atmosphere in a room and cleanse away any negativity left behind by difficult conversations, arguments or unkindness. Here's how:

1   Sit comfortably in the room and switch on Reiki.

2   Channel Reiki out of your hands and visualize it filling the room with a pure bright light.

3   Continue to do this until you feel the atmosphere in the room become lighter and welcoming.

You can also do a similar exercise to protect your space.

1   Stand at the entrance to a room, home or whatever space you wish to protect.

2   Hold your palms out in front of you.

3   Channel Reiki and visualize it creating a barrier across the entrance. Imagine a shield or strong metal door, or whatever symbolizes protection to you. Like the Reiki bubble (learn this on page 75), this wall of Reiki will let in positivity and love and keep out negativity.

REIKI AFFIRMATIONS

Affirmations are statements supporting what you want to be true. The law of attraction means that like attracts like, so whatever thoughts you send out will be reflected back to you as real situations in your life. If you state something to be true (affirm it), believe it and act like it is true, you will be more likely to bring that into reality. Repeating positive affirmations can help align your energy with the energy you wish to attract. You can use affirmations to help you become a clearer Reiki channel and also to help you to live out the Reiki principles.

Affirmations are most effective when they are in the present tense, worded as though they are happening now and accompanied by gratitude that they are a reality.

Here are some affirmations that might help you on your Reiki journey:

- I am an open and pure Reiki channel
- I am grateful for Reiki's presence in my life
- Reiki blessings pour into my life

- I am free from worry
- I am calm, I am positive
- I show respect to all living things
- I am blessed with wonderful people in my life
- I am honest and open
- I am grateful
- Reiki eases my pain
- Reiki calms my mind
- I easily step into the flow of Reiki

To help remember your chosen affirmations, write them on notes and stick them onto your mirror, noticeboard or fridge door. You could also set them as an alert on your phone or as the background image on your home screen. Affirmations work best when they are from the heart and feel aligned to the truth of your soul.

REIKI MEDITATION FOR AFFIRMATIONS

Self-Reiki while meditating on an affirmation can really help to strengthen that thought. Here's a simple but effective meditation for affirmations.

1   Sit or lie comfortably, close your eyes and take three deep breaths.

2   Ground yourself by connecting to the earth in whichever way suits you.

3   Place one hand across your brow chakra (forehead) and the other behind your head at the base of your head/nape of your neck.

4   Switch Reiki on and start channelling it into your head.

5   Think of an affirmation that you would like to charge and strengthen with Reiki. Remember to keep it in the present tense and positive.

6   Repeat your affirmation while letting Reiki flow into your mind, empowering the thought.

7   Continue this meditation for as long as you wish.

YOU DON'T
BECOME WHAT
YOU WANT, YOU
BECOME WHAT
YOU BELIEVE.

OPRAH WINFREY

REIKI BOX

A Reiki box is a great way of sending energy to the things you can't physically touch, such as the mental, emotional and spiritual areas of your life. The box allows you to focus Reiki energy and your positive intentions onto its contents. You can use it to send healing Reiki energy to any non-physical concerns in your life, such as mental well-being, relationships and work problems. Here's how...

Find yourself a small box that you can either hold in your hands or comfortably place one hand over. You can use a wooden box, cardboard gift box, old match box, empty tin or anything you feel drawn to. Decorating it yourself can give you the therapeutic benefits of being creative, as well as make it truly your own, but you don't have to.

Hold the box in your hands for a few minutes and state your intention that this is your Reiki box. Write any aspects of your life that you would like to send Reiki to on small slips of paper. You don't have to go into detail. Just a few words will be fine – something like "my relationship", "confidence" or "work", for example.

Separating your thoughts out to one thought per piece of paper can help bring order, while writing out concerns can make you feel as though you are releasing them from your mind, giving you space to think clearly. Place the slips one at a time into your Reiki box, visualizing good outcomes for each aspect as you do.

Now, whenever you wish to send Reiki to these aspects of your life, you can hold your Reiki box in your hands and switch on Reiki, channelling energy out of your hands into the box. Say in your mind that the healing Reiki energy will be sent to all the things inside, soothing and bringing positive change. You can do this daily or just whenever you feel the need. Using your Reiki box can help you feel you can take a positive action over an issue you might otherwise feel powerless over.

If you decide to do Reiki training, you will learn more about how to send Reiki through space and time to other people and situations, but this method is a very effective way of Reiki healing for your own life.

Trust Reiki,

all is well

A QUICK REIKI BOOST

If you find yourself feeling tired during the day, a quick and simple self-Reiki treatment can be just as effective as a nap, if not more so. This Reiki boost is great, as it only uses one hand position and gives you the energy you need to feel rejuvenated and be able to continue on with your day.

1   Sit or lie down and relax in a quiet spot.

2   Place one hand over your solar plexus (the centre of your body, just below your chest), and the other hand just below it (the little finger of your second hand will probably fall somewhere just above your navel).

3   Switch on Reiki and channel it into your body through your hands and relax.

4   Stay in this position for 10–15 minutes if possible. If you don't have much time, that's fine. Some self-Reiki is better than none!

REIKI TRAINING

This book has given you everything you need to give yourself Reiki. However, there are many Reiki secrets that are only divulged from a master to their student. If you have enjoyed learning self-Reiki and using the ideas in this book, consider finding a Reiki master (make sure you find someone reputable by looking at the recommended reading section at the end of this book) and learning more. As you go through the levels of training, you will learn "distance Reiki," as well as symbols and sounds that will help you fine-tune the frequency and intention of Reiki energy. You will also receive certification that shows your Reiki lineage tracing back to Mikao Usui.

Level one gives you your first attunements and empowerments, and you'll learn the history of Reiki, the concept of it, methods and hand positions. Most of this information is found in this book, but don't underestimate the benefits of learning from an experienced master. Once you have completed level one, you can progress to level two, where you'll learn how to treat other people both in person and from a distance. This is the level required to become insured and practise professionally. Level three is the master level, after which you will be able to teach Reiki to others. Some masters split the levels differently, so it's worth doing your research before you begin. Choose a Reiki master who you feel comfortable with and take your time between levels to really get to know the energy flow and how it feels for you before you move on to the next level. There is no end to learning Reiki. As you grow and evolve, Reiki reveals new and wonderful parts of itself to you. Even people who have been masters for many years still have new, beautiful Reiki experiences.

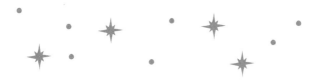

DO NOT WORRY.

DO NOT BE ANGRY.

BE HONEST.

BE GRATEFUL.

BE KIND.

BE A CLEAR CHANNEL

There are some things that can affect your ability to be a clear channel for Reiki. Here's how to help keep your channel clear:

1 Avoid too much alcohol

2 Eat healthily

3 Move your body regularly. This can be any movement, such as dancing, stretching or walking

4 Avoid drugs

5 Don't smoke

6 Be mindful and present

7 Take time to relax

8 Hold a good posture and breathe well

9 Get enough sleep

10 Avoid negativity

11 Use crystals (research and use your intuition to choose ones that work for you)

12 Meditate regularly

13 Maintain well-balanced chakras

14 Connect to the source of Reiki regularly

REIKI AS A SPIRITUAL PRACTICE

Reiki is a holistic complementary therapy and can be used to ease physical discomfort, emotional issues and boost well-being, but it can also be used as a spiritual practice.

Connecting to Reiki involves trust in a higher power or source. The act of connecting to the source of Reiki, no matter what you believe it is, can be thought of as an act of faith.

Regular self-Reiki, along with embracing the Reiki principles, is often considered a spiritual practice, as it encourages spiritual experiences and growth. Because Reiki is universal, it can be used alongside any other spiritual disciplines or faiths. You might like to consider whether you are only using Reiki for its therapeutic benefits (which is fine) or if you would like to develop your own spiritual practice.

If you already have religious or spiritual observances, you could add Reiki to enrich your practice. Or you could start with Reiki and explore whether you would like to include elements of religious traditions over time. Be aware that it's important to be respectful and mindful when using traditions and cultural practices that aren't your own. While Reiki is universal, many cultures have had to fight for the right to practise their faith, and it's a complicated and sensitive area. Think about why you are drawn to these practices and how you will be respectful of their origins and culture.

Building your own unique spiritual path is enriching and empowering. Reiki can be a beautiful foundation for that. A practice of daily self-Reiki sessions and repetition of the Reiki principles is a simple but effective way to nourish yourself spiritually and can be supplemented with Hatsu Rei Ho (page 80), a Reiki box (page 112) and/or meditations as you feel necessary.

Each person's experience of Reiki is unique to themselves. Don't judge yourself and your Reiki journey by how other people do it. Keep an open mind and heart – trust your instincts and Reiki's intelligence to guide you.

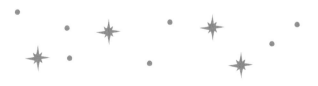

BE MORE REIKI

Look for daily opportunities to act out Reiki principles. Here's how:

- Take a deep breath and think calmly in difficult situations

- Avoid negative conversations that can spiral into bemoaning the state of the world

- Offer constructive suggestions to others who are worrying

- Give comfort and reassurance to worriers

- Talk about positive, uplifting stories you have heard

- Take a deep breath and count to ten instead of reacting in anger

- If someone annoys you, try to look at their point of view or motives

- Channel anger into positive action – vote, campaign or write to leaders

- Spread the word about positive change and how others can get involved

- Let the little stuff go
- Take a moment to listen to someone; let them know you have heard them
- Smile and make eye contact with people
- Pay compliments to strangers
- Work on being open and accepting of others
- Be helpful in small ways, such as opening doors for people
- Look at ways you can help the environment
- Support your local community
- Speak your truth kindly
- Look at ways to improve your work situation – not just for you but also for colleagues
- Make lifestyle changes that align with your beliefs, such as recycling more or buying environmentally friendly products
- Thank people, no matter how small their deed
- Keep a gratitude journal
- Tell people what it is about them that you are grateful for

- List three things every day that you are thankful for

- Tell people when they have made a positive difference to your day

- Repeat the Reiki principles every day to keep them fresh in your mind

Of course, this is a short list – the ways to embrace the Reiki principles are endless.

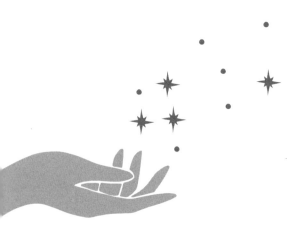

FAREWELL

You have now discovered and stepped into the flow of the pure, loving energy that is Reiki. You have gained a powerful and yet gentle tool for healing yourself physically, mentally, emotionally and spiritually and to create positive change in your life. You may have made Reiki your new spiritual practice or added it to an existing one. You might even go on to train and treat others.

Accept Reiki with respect and awe as the precious gift it is and enjoy its healing presence in your life.

This is just the first step. From now on, Reiki will always be there for you when you turn to it. Whether you use Reiki daily, weekly or just every now and then, no matter how long it's been since you last used it, it's always there, unconditional, strong and true. Just stay open and trust.

Remember: Just for today, set aside worry and anger, respect all living things, be true to yourself and feel gratitude for all life's blessings.

May Reiki flow through you, heal you, protect you and bring you peace, love and joy.

FURTHER READING

Reiki Rays: www.reikirays.com
The Reiki Healing Association:
  www.reikihealingassociation.com
The UK Reiki Federation: www.reikifed.co.uk
The Reiki Association: www.reikiassociation.net

Reiki Healing and Harmony Through the Hands
Tanmaya Honervogt
Gaia Books

*The Reiki Manual: A Training Guide for Reiki
Students, Practitioners and Masters*
Penelope Quest
Piatkus

*Reiki For Beginners: Mastering Natural Healing
Techniques*
David Vennells
Llewellyn Publications

Reiki and the Seven Chakras
Richard Ellis
Vermillion

The Little Book of Chakras
Elsie Wild
Summersdale Publishers Ltd

IMAGE CREDITS

Sun icon © Marish/Shutterstock.com
Textured gradient background ©
Alex Tihonovs/Shutterstock.com
p.22 © DeoSum/Shutterstock.com
pp.64–69, 82 – line drawings by Agnes Graves
All other illustrations © knstartstudio/Shutterstock.com

Have you enjoyed this book?
If so, find us on Facebook at **Summersdale Publishers**, on Twitter at **@Summersdale** and on Instagram at **@summersdalebooks** and get in touch. We'd love to hear from you!

www.summersdale.com